Jorge Fernando Rebouças Lessa
Maria Célia Brangioni
Thiago Xavier Corrêa

Treatment of zolpidem dependence: a review of clinical cases

Jorge Fernando Rebouças Lessa
Maria Célia Brangioni
Thiago Xavier Corrêa

Treatment of zolpidem dependence: a review of clinical cases

Monograph presented to conclude the Medical Residency Programme in Psychiatry at HUB

ScienciaScripts

Cover image: www.ingimage.com

This book is a translation from the original published under ISBN 978-613-9-66050-6.

Publisher:
Sciencia Scripts
is a trademark of
Dodo Books Indian Ocean Ltd. and OmniScriptum S.R.L publishing group

120 High Road, East Finchley, London, N2 9ED, United Kingdom
Str. Armeneasca 28/1, office 1, Chisinau MD-2012, Republic of Moldova, Europe
Printed at: see last page
ISBN: 978-620-7-98216-5

ACKNOWLEDGEMENTS

To the friends and companions of this journey, Dr Thiago Xavier, Dr Macei, Dr Tallita Dantas, Dr Diana, Dr Deborah, who often shared the work, shared experiences and were essential in this journey.

To the resident doctors of the Medical Residency Programmes (PRM) of the Hospital e Base do Distrito Federal, Hospital das Forças Armadas for their support at all times.

To all the preceptors at the Hospital São Vicente de Paulo for all their dedication in welcoming us, especially Dr Jussane for her professional example.

To Dr Fabiano for giving up his time and donating his knowledge and work for the success of this medical residency.

To Dr Thais Sarmento, Dr Camila Herculano, Dr Josie Anne for having made all the difference with their dedication, uprightness and companionship.

Dr Maria Célia for guiding us so patiently in this and other work we have done.

To my beloved wife for encouraging me in my weakest moments and always optimistically filling me with hope for the future.

To my children for cheering me up and inspiring me to keep going.

"And though I had the gift of prophecy, and knew all mysteries and all knowledge, and though I had all faith, so that I could move mountains, and had not love, I should be nothing." Paul of Tarsus 1 Corinthians 13:2

SUMMARY

Introduction:

Zolpidem is a non-benzodiazepine hypnotic used to treat insomnia, which selectively binds to the alpha unit of GABA receptors. Therapeutic doses range from 5mg to 10mg a day. Continuous use, as well as doses above those reported, are associated with memory loss, tolerance, dependence and withdrawal syndrome. The latter is associated with anxiety symptoms, sleep disorders, autonomic dysfunction and seizures.

Objectives:

To analyse 40 clinical cases described in the literature as a series of cases of Zolpidem dependence and its treatment, as well as the presence of associated psychiatric pathologies.

Methods:

Search in the PUBMED database with the terms (("zolpidem") and ("pharmacodependence" or "abuse" or "dependence" or "dependency" or "addiction" or "reward" or "reward system" or "tolerance" or "withdrawal" or "abstinence")) on 24/08/2016. Only case reports with reference to the treatment of zolpidem dependence were selected.

Results:

We found 86 articles on clinical cases of zolpidem dependence or abuse. Of these, only 34 articles with 40 case reports referred to the treatment of zolpidem dependence, abuse or intoxication. The average age of this sample was 42.35 years; 21 (52.5%) were male and 19 (47.5) female. Some psychiatric comorbidity was reported in 35 (87.5%) cases, and in 1 neurological comorbidity (multiple sclerosis and paraspasticity). Of the psychiatric comorbidities, 54.2 per cent had other active chemical dependencies or had a history of chemical dependency; 34.3 per cent had depression; 11.4 per cent had anxiety; 8.5 per cent had bipolar mood disorder; 5.7 per cent had personality disorder. The doses of zolpidem used ranged from 30 to 2,000mg / day. Withdrawal symptoms were reported in 72.5 per cent of cases, of which 45.7 per cent had seizures. All those who had seizures were using a dose of 100mg or more of zolpidem daily. For the treatment of zolpidem dependence, the majority used benzodiazepines (67.5%), followed by zolpidem (42.1%), serotonin receptor inhibitors (SSRIs) (32.5%) and anticonvulsants (25%). But other drugs were also used to a lesser extent: atypical antipsychotics 12.5%, trazodone 10%; mirtazapine and flumazenil 7.5%; tricyclics 5%; baclofen, typical antipsychotics and anticholinesterases 2.5%. More than one drug was used in 70% of cases.

Conclusion:

Our study showed that benzodiazepines, zolpidem itself, SSRIs and anticonvulsants were used most frequently to treat this dependence. Controlled studies are needed to better understand zolpidem dependence, its association with psychiatric pathologies, and to develop specific treatment protocols.

Key words:

zolpidem, dependence, comorbidities, treatment.

SUMMARY

CHAPTER 1

INTRODUCTION

Benzodiazepines (BDZs) are still commonly prescribed for the short-term treatment of insomnia, but have gradually been replaced by Zolpidem due to its favourable pharmacokinetic profile, proven clinical efficacy, relative safety and good tolerability. These characteristics have contributed to its popularisation in clinical practice (Holm KJ, Goa KL., 2000).

Zolpidem is a non-benzodiazepine hypnotic that selectively binds to the alpha unit of GABA receptors. It is rapidly absorbed, reaching peak plasma concentration in 0.8 to 2.6 hours. Therapeutic doses range from 5 mg to 10 mg a day. Doses above this value are associated with sleep problems, memory loss and withdrawal syndrome. This is similar to that of BDZs, with anxiety symptoms, sleep disorders, autonomic dysfunction and seizures (Hwang TJ, Liappas IA, Tripodianakis J 2003). These data suggest that, at high doses, zolpidem is no longer selective, but also acts on GABA-A receptors containing the a2, a3 and a5 subunits and has pharmacodynamics and additive potential similar to BZDs. (Go der R *et al* 2001)

According to the International Statistical Classification of Diseases and Related Health Problems, ICD 10, (F13 - Mental and behavioural disorders due to the use of sedatives and hypnotics) the diagnostic criteria for dependence on psychoactive substances, including sedative hypnotics or anxiolytics, are generalised to any substance (attached). However, the Diagnostic and Statistical Manual of Mental Disorders - DSM V has taken particular care to characterise the disorders related to this dependence, which are listed below:

A problematic pattern of sedative, hypnotic or anxiolytic use, leading to clinically significant impairment or distress, manifested by at least two of the following criteria, occurring over a 12-month period:

1. Sedatives, hypnotics or anxiolytics are often consumed in larger quantities or for a longer period than intended.

2. There is a persistent desire or unsuccessful efforts to reduce or control the use of sedatives, hypnotics or anxiolytics.

3. A lot of time is spent on the activities required to obtain the sedative, hypnotic or anxiolytic, on using these substances or recovering from their effects.

4. Fissure or a strong desire or need to use the sedative, hypnotic or anxiolytic.

5. Recurrent use of sedatives, hypnotics or anxiolytics resulting in failure to fulfil important obligations at work, school or home (e.g. constant absences from work or low work performance related to the use of sedatives, hypnotics or anxiolytics; absences, suspensions or expulsions from school related to sedatives, hypnotics or anxiolytics; neglect of children or household chores).

6. Continued use of sedatives, hypnotics or anxiolytics despite persistent or recurrent social or interpersonal problems caused or exacerbated by the effects of these substances (e.g. arguments with the spouse about the consequences of intoxication; physical aggression).

7. Important social, professional or recreational activities are abandoned or reduced due to the use of sedatives, hypnotics or anxiolytics.

8. Recurrent use of sedatives, hypnotics or anxiolytics in situations where this poses a danger to physical integrity (e.g. driving vehicles or operating machinery during impairment due to the use of sedatives, hypnotics or anxiolytics).

9. The use of sedatives, hypnotics or anxiolytics is maintained despite the awareness of having a persistent or recurring physical or psychological

problem probably caused or exacerbated by these substances.

10. Tolerance, defined by any of the following aspects:

a. The need for progressively larger quantities of the sedative, hypnotic or anxiolytic to achieve intoxication or the desired effect.

b. Significantly less effect with continued use of the same amount of sedative, hypnotic or anxiolytic.

Note: This criterion is disregarded in individuals whose use of sedatives, hypnotics or anxiolytics is under medical supervision.

11. Abstinence, manifested by any of the following:

a. Withdrawal syndrome characteristic of sedatives, hypnotics or anxiolytics (see Criteria A and B of the set of criteria for withdrawal from sedatives, hypnotics or anxiolytics, p. 557-558). 13

b. Sedatives, hypnotics or anxiolytics (or a closely related substance such as alcohol) are consumed to relieve or avoid withdrawal symptoms.

Note: This criterion is disregarded in individuals whose use of sedatives, hypnotics or anxiolytics is under medical supervision. (DSM-V pg 550)

Criteria A and B

A. Cessation (or reduction) of prolonged use of sedatives, hypnotics or anxiolytics.

B. Two (or more) of the following symptoms, developed within several hours to a few days after cessation (or reduction) of the use of sedatives, hypnotics or anxiolytics described in Criterion A:

1. Autonomic hyperactivity (e.g. sweating or heart rate above 100 BPM).
2. Hands trembling.
3. Insomnia.
4. Nausea or vomiting.
5. Transient visual, tactile or auditory hallucinations or illusions.
6. Psychomotor agitation.

7. Anxiety.
8. Seizures of the grand mal type (DSM-V pages 557-558)

The 12-month prevalence of DSM-IV sedative, hypnotic or anxiolytic use disorder is estimated to be 0.3 per cent in the 12 to 17 age group and 0.2 per cent among adults aged 18 and over. Rates of DSM-IV disorder are slightly higher among adult males (0.3 per cent) than adult females, but from 12 to 17 years of age, the rate for girls (0.4 per cent) exceeds the rate for boys (0.2 per cent). The 12-month prevalence of DSM-IV disorder decreases with age and is highest between the ages of 18 and 29 (0.5 per cent) and lowest among individuals aged 65 and over (0.04 per cent).

The 12-month prevalence of sedative, hypnotic or anxiolytic use disorder varies from one racial/ethnic subgroup to another in the North American population. Among 12 to 17 year olds, rates are higher among whites (0.3%) than among African-Americans (0.2%), Hispanics (0.2%), Native Americans (0.1%) and Asian-Americans and Pacific Islanders (0.1%). Among adults, the 12-month prevalence is highest among American Indians and Alaska Natives (0.8%), with rates of 0.2% among African Americans, Whites and Hispanics and 0.1% among Asian Americans and Pacific Islanders (DSM-V page 553).

A study on addiction to non-benzodiazepine hypnotics concluded that Zolpidem is relatively safe when compared to benzodiazepines. The data revealed that among the 1,338,774,000 Zolpidem tablets prescribed between 2001 and 2002 in the USA, Europe and Japan, only 36 cases of pharmacodependence were reported in the period 1966 to 2002, through publications in the literature (G. Hajak et al). However, this study was funded by a pharmaceutical laboratory, which may have led to research bias and compromised the reliability of the results

The addictive potential of zolpidem was already being discussed in the

1990s (Evans SM et al, 1990). The results of observations on behavioural reinforcers in humans have shown that the abuse potential of Zolpidem is similar to that of benzodiazepines (Rush CR. 1998 // Evans SM, Funderburk FR, Griffiths RR. 1990).

Studies have examined the behavioural effects of Zolpidem in baboons. This medication caused excessive sedation, which reduced after 7 consecutive days of use. In addition, exchanging the substance for a placebo produced withdrawal syndrome. The results were similar to those found with the use of benzodiazepines and are divergent from studies with rodents. (Griffiths RR, Sannerud CA, Ator NA, Brady JV. 1992 //Weerts EM, Griffiths RR. 1998)

Initial studies in rodents revealed no evidence of tolerance to the sedative effect or physical dependence, assessed by the absence of withdrawal symptoms after prolonged administration and discontinuation of the drug, unlike benzodiazepines. (Elliot EE, White JM. 2000; Perrault G, Morei E, Sanger DJ, Zivkovic B. 1992) In contrast, there is complete tolerance to the hypothermic and muscle relaxant effects in rodents after 8 days of treatment (in rodents, zolpidem has three effects: hypothermic, muscle relaxant and sedative) (Elliot EE, White JM. 2000).

A meta-analysis of 137 studies found no evidence of tolerance of the Zolpidem. However, this same study showed a higher risk of rebound insomnia compared to placebo (Soldatos CR, Dikeos DG, Whitehead A. 1999) 15

Lemoine *et* al in 1995 reported withdrawal syndrome after 3 months of treatment with zolpidem 10 mg / day

In a study carried out to assess the presence or absence of rebound insomnia with zolpidem after 28 days of treatment, controlled by two groups, one placebo and the other by triazolam 0.5 mg (double the recommended dose), known to produce rebound insomnia, showed that after 4 weeks the level of efficacy decreased for both drugs. (Ware JC, Walsh JK, Scharf MB,

Roehrs T, Roth T, Vogel GW. 1997). This result is similar to the one found by Voderholzer *et al* in 2001, except that the subjects were healthy.

In 2009, another study showed that the use of therapeutic doses of zolpidem promotes an acute reduction in GABA levels in the thalamic region of healthy individuals without a history of any psychiatric disorder. (Licata, Stephanie et al, 2009) In another study, Goddard *et al.* in 2004, showed a reduction in GABA levels in a similar proportion in the occipital cortex after the administration of clonazepam.

Studies in healthy volunteers showed a reduction in regional cerebral blood flow of approximately 20 per cent (Matthew et al., 1995, Veselis et al 1997) and a 23 per cent reduction in glucose metabolism (Volkow et al 1995; Wang et al. 1996) after administration of benzodiazepines. Similarly, local cerebral glucose metabolism was reduced in subcortical areas when participants were given zolpidem (Gillin et al., 1996). These results suggest that the thalamus is a region of action for benzodiazepines and also for non-benzodiazepine hypnotics such as zolpidem.

The results of these studies suggest a similarity in action profile between benzodiazepines and zolpidem.

France has its own system for assessing the addictive potential of psychoactive medications: Centre for Evaluation and Information on Pharmacodependence (CEIP) (C. Victorri-Vigneau *et al.* 2014). In 2001, French health authorities (National Agency for Medicines and Health Products Safety-ANSM) commissioned an official CEIP study to assess the addictive potential of zolpidem. (C. Victorri-Vigneau *et al.* 2007) The results showed that zolpidem has a high potential for abuse and identified two groups of users: the first who experienced euphoria, exaltation and obtained anxiolytic but not hypnotic effects; another group of patients who used the medication for sedative purposes to treat insomnia. (C. Victorri-Vigneau *et al.* 2007)

Therefore, in 2014, information about Zolpidem was modified, including the following sentence on the product: "The pharmacodependence may materialise even at therapeutic doses, and/or for subjects who do not show an individualised risk factor (Une pharmacodépendance peut survenir à doses thérapeutiques et/ou chez des patients sans facteur de risque individualisé)." (Pharmacodependence can occur even at therapeutic doses and/or for subjects who do not show an individualised risk factor). http://base- donnees-publique.medicaments.gouv.fr/index.php#result (C. Victorri-Vigneau *et al.* 2014)

The World Health Organisation (WHO) considered that the frequency of Zolpidem dependence is similar to that of benzodiazepines. In 2002, Zolpidem was transferred to "Schedule IV of the 1971 Convention", relating to the classification of potential dependence on the psychotropic drug. The aim of this convention is to control both the traffic in and abuse of psychotropic drugs. (LRP. Dépendance aux hypnotiques: zolpidem et zopiclone aussi. Rev Prescr 2002; 20: 675-6. // LRP. Zolpidem: classed as a psychotropic drug at risk of abuse. Rev Prescr 2002; 22: 819).

CHAPTER 2

OBJECTIVES

To analyse the case reports of zolpidem dependence in the PUBMED database that refer to the treatment of zolpidem intoxication and/or dependence.

To analyse the presence of psychiatric comorbidities associated with zolpidem dependence.

To evaluate the treatment administered to zolpidem-dependent patients and thus be able to gather information that could suggest a direction for clinical practice in the treatment of zolpidem dependence.

CHAPTER 3

METHODOLOGY

DESIGN

A secondary, observational study of the systematic literature review type, with critical analysis of the results using case reports for its elaboration. This scientific method is considered to be explicit and reproducible, demonstrating a better level of evidence for decision-making.

This work involved two researchers who created a research protocol based on the topic of interest and the inclusion and exclusion criteria. The researchers independently assessed the methodological quality of each article, checked the accuracy of the results and extracted the data to be organised in table format.

SELECTION OF ARTICLES

The search was carried out in the PubMed electronic database, with no restrictions on language or year of publication, using the term "zolpidem" combined with "pharmacodependence", "abuse", "dependence", "addiction", "reward", "reward system", "tolerance", "withdrawal" and "abstinence". Finally, the 467 articles were filtered to select only case reports.

A total of 86 articles were found on 24/08/2016. The researchers assessed the titles and abstracts in accordance with the predetermined inclusion and exclusion criteria, and in cases of doubt, the texts were analysed in full.

INCLUSION CRITERIA

Original case report or series;

Presence of information on the clinical management of Zolpidem addiction;

No language limitations;

EXCLUSION CRITERIA

Other studies.

DATA EXTRACTION

For each case, the authors extracted information on age, gender, presence of psychiatric comorbidity, initial and final dose of zolpidem, withdrawal symptoms, time of use, medications used to treat zolpidem dependence and treatment setting and regime (table attached).

CHAPTER 4

RESULTS

A total of 86 articles on clinical cases of zolpidem dependence were found, of which only 34, with 40 case reports, referred to the treatment of zolpidem dependence. The average age found in the cases studied was 42.35 years; 21 (52.5%) cases were male and 19 (47.5%) were female (Figure I).

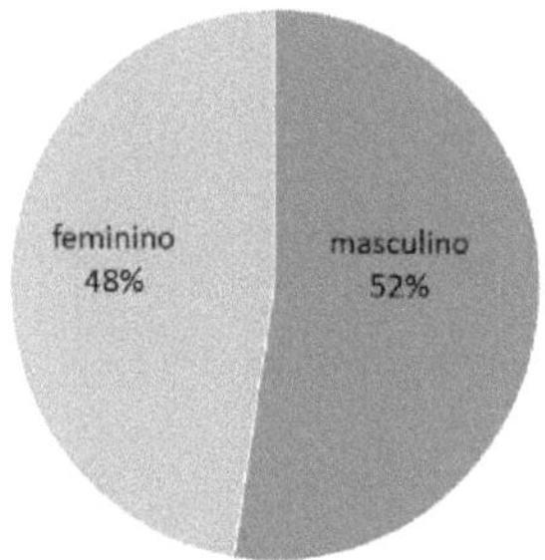

Figura I: Gender distribution of the sample

In 35 (87.5%) cases some psychiatric comorbidity was reported, and 1 (2.5%) had a neurological comorbidity (multiple sclerosis and paraspasticity). Of the psychiatric comorbidities, 54.2% had other active chemical dependencies or had a history of chemical dependency; 34.3% had depression; 11.4% had anxiety; 8.5% had bipolar mood disorder; 5.7% had personality disorder (Figure II).

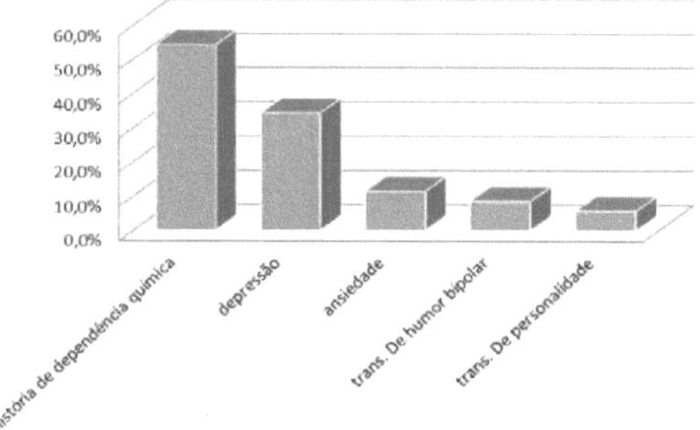

Figura II: psychiatric comorbidities associated with zolpidem dependence

The doses of zolpidem used ranged from 30 to 2,000mg / day.

In 28 (70 per cent) cases the time of use of zolpidem was recorded, in 2 (5 per cent) cases the time of use was identified as more than 2 months, the rest, 26 (95 per cent) cases, the time of use ranged from 6 months to 15 years.

Withdrawal symptoms were reported in 72.5 per cent of cases, of which 45.7 per cent had seizures when attempting to reduce the dose. In these cases, the patients were taking a daily dose of 100mg or more of zolpidem.

Several classes of drug have been used to treat zolpidem dependence. We can highlight benzodiazepines (67.5%), zolpidem itself (42.1%), serotonin receptor inhibitors (SSRIs) (32.5%) and anticonvulsants (25%). In the cases where zolpidem was used (42.1%), 56.25% of them were gradually reduced, and 43.75% were cross-treated with other drugs. (Figure III) Other drugs were also used: atypical antipsychotics in 5 cases (12.5%), trazodone in 4 cases (10%); mirtazapine and flumazenil both in 3 cases (7.5%); tricyclics in 2 cases (5%); baclofen, typical antipsychotics and anticholinesterases in 1 case each (2.5%). (Figure III)

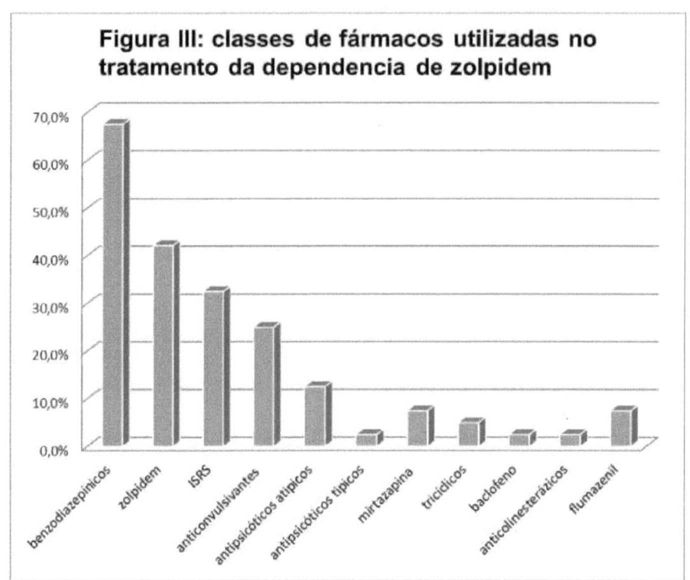

Figura III: classes de fármacos utilizadas no tratamento da dependencia de zolpidem

Two or more medications were used in 28 (70%) of the cases.

In 12 (30 per cent) of the cases reported, treatment was monotherapy, of which 6 (50 per cent) used benzodiazepines, 3 (25 per cent) used SSRIs, 2 (16.66 per cent) used zolpidem itself; divalproate was

used as monotherapy in only 1 (8.33 per cent) case.

There was a preference for abruptly withdrawing zolpidem in 22 (57.9%) cases. In 9 (22.5%) cases, treatment was carried out with a gradual reduction in the dose of zolpidem and in 7 (17.5%) cases there was a cross-over regime with another medication. In 2 (5%) cases there was no information on the treatment regimen.

The treatment environment was reported in 32 (80%) cases, of which 27 (84.375%) were in a hospital environment, 2 (6.25%) in an outpatient environment and 3 (9.375%) in both (Figure IV).

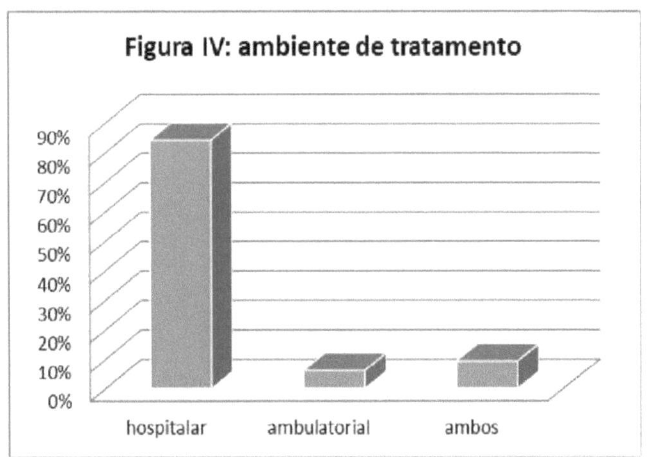

There was a description of the duration of treatment for zolpidem dependence in 17 (42.5%) cases, of which 14 (82.3%) were inpatient, 1 (5.9%) outpatient and 2 (5%), whose time was stated in the article, made no reference to the place of treatment. In all cases, the length of stay ranged from 3 days to 3 months, with the longest period of hospitalisation reported being 2 months. However, in the majority of admissions, 12 (70.5%) were hospitalised for detoxification for less than 3 weeks.

In only 3 (7.5%) cases was adjuvant psychotherapy used.

CHAPTER 5

DISCUSSION

At the time of data collection for this study, there was no established therapeutic protocol in the literature for the treatment of zolpidem dependence. One of the withdrawal symptoms of considerable severity and frequency observed in the case reports is seizures. These should attract the attention and care of health professionals when prescribing zolpidem and especially when reducing or discontinuing this medication.

Of the medications available in the therapeutic arsenal, benzodiazepines, zolpidem itself (in gradual reduction or cross-exchange), SSRIs and anticonvulsants were used preferentially, perhaps due to the relative safety of these drugs.

The action of benzodiazepines on GABA receptors, as well as their anticonvulsant effect, suggests an explanation for the high frequency of their use for the treatment of zolpidem dependence in our study.

Strategies have been established for the detoxification of high-dose short half-life BZDs, following two principles: gradually decreasing and using equivalent doses of long-acting BZDs as substitutes (Alexander B, 1991; Ashton H, 2005). However, it is uncertain whether this treatment strategy can also be applied to zolpidem.

Scatton et al, in 1986, showed that zolpidem reduces serotonin synthesis in the hippocampus, striatum and frontal cortex. Koyama et al in 1999 showed that activation of pre-synaptic serotonin receptors occurs to inhibit synaptic release of GABA. Furthermore, the serotonergic system lacks functional specialisation and interacts with cholinergic, glutamatergic, dopaminergic and also gabaergic systems, playing a role in a wide variety of behaviours (Buhot *et al.,* 2000). This information makes up the serotonergic hypothesis proposed by Liappas *et al.* in 2003 to explain the efficacy of selective serotonin receptor inhibitors in the treatment of zolpidem dependence.

The data from this study is in line with the literature on the subject, which deals with the frequent presence of psychiatric comorbidities in drug addiction in general (Alves, Kessler, & Ratto, 2004; Scheffer, Pasa, & de Almeida, 2010; Zaleski et al., 2006). They also show an association between zolpidem dependence and other psychiatric disorders and suggest that the presence of psychiatric comorbidity may be a risk factor for zolpidem dependence, since the prescription of zolpidem for the treatment of insomnia associated with psychiatric disorders has replaced the prescription of benzodiazepines for this purpose (Holm KJ, Goa KL., 2000). This reinforces the need for greater caution in prescribing this substance.

The significant presence of psychiatric comorbidities, described in 87.5% of the cases analysed, the lack of clinical studies aimed at treating zolpidem dependence, the need to contain clinical symptoms associated with the suspension of this drug and/or psychiatric symptoms of dependent patients during hospital stays, or the complexity of this dependence, whose withdrawal symptoms are quite varied, some of which are quite serious, such as seizures and psychotic symptoms, and others which are not as serious but have great potential for discomfort for the patient, such as insomnia and anxiety attacks, suggest a possible explanation for the high presence, in 70 per cent of the cases studied, of the use of more than one drug in the treatment.

It is important to emphasise that patients with a history and/or activity of other chemical dependencies, as seen in this study (54.2%), suggest that care should be taken when prescribing zolpidem to these patients.

It should be noted that non-pharmacological intervention as an adjunct, in this case psychotherapy, was not very common in the study. And given the existence in the scientific literature of evidence that sufficiently confirms its importance in the treatment of psychiatric disorders, drug addiction and insomnia, this therapeutic technique could indeed help in the treatment of zolpidem addiction if it were made more widely available.

The data on the treatment environment follows the trend of other addictions, which, in the case of severe intoxication or moderate to severe withdrawal syndrome, are recommended to be treated in a general hospital, given the high risk of clinical complications. (Ronaldo Laranjeira et al, Chemical dependency prevention, treatment and public policies 2011)

Several randomised double-blind studies have shown that sudden discontinuation of zolpidem treatment after 2 to 4 weeks was not associated with withdrawal symptoms, but the dosage in these controlled studies was within the normal recommended range (Holm KJ *et al* 2000; Vartzopoulos D *et al* 2000).

However, zolpidem has similar physiological and psychological reinforcing effects and abuse potential to benzodiazepines (Toner LC *et al* 2000).

In the literature there are 3 reports of intravenous zolpidem abuse, 2 of which are associated with dependence on other injectable drugs (Benyamina, Amine et al, 2007; Kao, Ching-Ling et al 2004). The major risk of this route of administration is the formation of thrombi due to the presence of cellulose microcrystals in the formulation of zolpidem tablets (Kao, Ching-Ling *et al* 2004).

CHAPTER 6

CONCLUSION

The data from this study, although scarce, provides us with reflections on the need for medical practice in the treatment of Zolpidem dependence. It is important that the doctor, when confirming a possible case of inappropriate use and/or dependence on Zolpidem, offers the patient treatment, preferably in two stages:

1ª - Outpatient or short-term inpatient detox, depending on the severity of the condition. In this situation, in a hospital environment, we suggest trying sudden withdrawal from zolpidem, and prescribing drugs with a sedative effect and the potential to control or prevent possible seizures, in situations where the doses of zolpidem used are high, and to ease the withdrawal symptoms that may be present. In cases of outpatient treatment, we suggest gradual withdrawal of zolpidem.

2ª - Outpatient follow-up to continue specific treatment for zolpidem dependence and any associated psychiatric comorbidities. Above all, the use of sedative medication, if necessary, without the potential for dependence.

The withdrawal symptoms observed immediately after abrupt discontinuation of zolpidem, described in the clinical cases included in this study, were: autonomic hyperactivity, tremors, insomnia, nausea and vomiting, alterations in sensory perception, paranoid symptoms, psychomotor agitation, anxiety and convulsive crises. They are compatible with the symptoms of withdrawal from sedatives, anxiolytics or hypnotics described in the DSM-V.

However, there is still a lot to know about zolpidem dependence, in terms of the specific psychopathological description, the description of the specific withdrawal syndrome and in relation to the specific treatment.

It is necessary to expand therapeutic techniques associated with pharmacotherapy, such as cognitive behavioural psychotherapy, motivational techniques and relapse prevention, since chemical dependency is a complex and multifaceted disorder, and zolpidem dependency is no exception.

However, controlled research is needed to better understand this addiction, its psychopathological manifestations, its association with psychiatric comorbidities, and above all to develop treatment protocols.

CHAPTER 7

BIBLIOGRAPHY

- Hwang TJ, Ni HC, Chen HC, Lin YT, Liao SC. **Risk predictors for hypnosedative-related complex sleep behaviours: a retrospective, cross-sectional pilot study. J** Clin Psychiatry 2010;71:1331-5.

- Liappas IA, Malitas PN, Dimopoulos NP, et al. **Zolpidem dependence case series: possible neurobiological mechanisms and clinical management. J** Psychopharmacol 2003;17:131-5.

- Hajak. G.; Muller, W. E.; Wittchen, H. U.; Pittrow, D.; Kirch,W; **.Abuse and dependence potential for the non-benzodiazepine hypnotics zolpidem and zopiclone: a review of case reports and epidemiological data.** Addiction, 98, 1371-1378

- Tripodianakis J, Potagas C, Papageorgiou P, Lazaridou M, Matikas N. **Zolpidem- related epileptic seizures: a case report.** Eur Psychiatry 2003; 18:140-1.

- Evans SM, Funderburk FR, Griffiths RR (1990) **Zolpidem and triazolam in humans: behavioural and subjective effects and abuse liability.** J Pharmacol Exp Ther 255:1246-1255

- Licata, Stephanie C., Jensen. J. Eric, Penetar, David M., Prescot, Andrew P., Lukas, Scott E., Renshaw, Perry F.; **A therapeutic dose of zolpidem reduces thalamic GABA in healthy volunteers: a proton MRS study at 4 T** Psychopharmacology (2009) 203:819-829

- Matthew E, Andreason P, Pettigrew K, Carson RE, Herscovitch P, Cohen R, King C, Johanson CE, Greenblatt DJ, Paul SM (1995) **Benzodiazepine receptors mediate regional blood flow changes in the living human brain.**

Proc Natl Acad Sei U S A 92:2775-2779

- Veselis RA, Reinsel RA, Beattie BJ, Mawlawi OR, Feshchenko VA, DiResta GR, Larson SM, Blasberg RG (1997) **Midazolam changes cerebral blood flow in discrete brain regions: an H2 (15)0 positron emission tomography study.** Anaesthesiology 87:1106-1117

- Volkow ND, Wang GJ, Hitzemann R, Fowler JS, Pappas N, Lowrimore P, Burr G, Pascani K, Overall J, Wolf AP (1995) **Depression of thalamic metabolism by lorazepam is associated with sleepiness.** Neuropsychopharmacology 12:123-132

- Wang GJ, Volkow ND, Overall J, Hitzemann RJ, Pappas N, Pascani K, Fowler JS (1996) **Reproducibility of regional brain metabolic responses to lorazepam.** J Nucl Med 37:1609-1613

- Gillin JC, Buchsbaum MS, Valladares-Neto DC, Hong CC-H, Hazlett E, Langer SZ, Wu J (1996) **Effects of zolpidem on local cerebral glucose metabolism during non-REM sleep in normal volunteers: a positron emission tomography study.** Neuropsycho-pharmacology 15:302-313

- C. Victorri-Vigneau et al. **An Update on Zolpidem Abuse and Dependence.** Journal of Addictive Diseases, 33:15-23, 2014

- C. Victorri-Vigneau et al. **Evidence of zolpidem abuse and dependence.** Br J Clin Pharmacol 2007

- Holm KJ, Goa KL. **Zolpidem: an update of its pharmacology, therapeutic efficacy and tolerability in the treatment of insomnia.** Drugs 2000; 59: 865-89.

- Ware JC, Walsh JK, Scharf MB, Roehrs T, Roth T, Vogel GW. **Minimal rebound insomnia after treatment with 10 mg zolpidem.** Clin Neuropharmacol 1997; 20: 116-25

- Voderholzer U, Riemann D, Hornyak M, Backhaus J, Feige B, Berger M, Hohagen **F. A double-blind, randomised and placebo-controlled study on the polysomnographic withdrawal effects of zopiclone, zolpidem and triazolam in healthy subjects.** EurArch Psychiatry Clin Neurosci 2001; 251: 117-23

- Lemoine P, Allain H, Janus C. **Gradual withdrawal of zopiclone (7.5 mg) and zolpidem (10 mg) in insomniacs treated for at least 3 months.** Eur Psychiatry 1995; 10(SuppL 3): 161s-165s

- Perrault G, Morei E, Sanger DJ, Zivkovic B. **Lack of tolerance and physical dependence upon repeated treatment with the novel hypnotic zolpidem.** J Pharmacol Exp Ther 1992; 263: 298-303.

- Griffiths RR, Sannerud CA, Ator NA, Brady JV. **Zolpidem behavioural pharmacology in baboons: self-injection, discrimination, tolerance and withdrawal.** J Pharmacol Exp Ther 1992; 260: 1199-208.

- Weerts EM, Griffiths RR. **Zolpidem self-injection with concurrent physical dependence under conditions of long-term continuous availability in baboons.** Behav Pharmacol 1998; 9: 285-97.

- Rush CR. **Behavioural pharmacology of zolpidem relative to benzodiazepines: a review.** Pharmacol Biochem Behav 1998; 61: 256-69.

- Scatton 6, Claustre Y, Dennis T, Nishikawa T (1986) **Zolpidem, a novel nonbenzodiazepine hypnotic. II. Effects on cerebellar cCMP and cerebral monoarnines.** J Pharm Exp Ther 237: 659-665.

- Koyama S, Kubo C, Rhee IS, Akaike N (1999) **Presynaptic serotonergic inhibition of GABAergic synaptic transmission in mechanically dissociated rat basolateral amygdala neurons.** J Physiol 51 8: 525-538.

- Buhot M, Martin 5, Segu L (2000) **Role of serotonin in memory**

impairment. Ann Med 32:210-221.

- Alexander B, Perry PJ. **Detoxification from benzodiazepines: schedules and strategies.** J Subst Abuse Treat 1991;8:9-17.

- Ashton H. **The diagnosis and management of benzodiazepine dependence.** Curr Opin Psychiatry 2005;18:249-55.

- Holm KJ & Goa KL. **Zolpidem: An update of its pharmacology, therapeutic efficacy and tolerability in the treatment of insomnia.** Drugs 2000; 59: 865-889.

- Vartzopoulos D, Bozikas V , Phocas C, Karavatos A & Kaprinis G. **Dependence on zolpidem in high dose.** IntClin Psychopharmacol 2000; 15: 181-182.

- Toner LC, Tsambiras BM, Catalano G, Catalano MC & Cooper DS. **Central nervous system side effects associated with zolpidem treatment.** Clin Neuropharmacol 2000; 23: 54-58.

- Go der R, Treskov V, Burmester J, Aldenhoff JB, Hinze-Selch D. Zolpidem: **The risk of tolerance and dependence according to case reports, systematic**

studies and recent molecular biological data. Fortschr Neurol Psychiatr. 2001;69:592-596

- Pick CG, Chernes Y, Rigai T, Rice KC, Schreiber S. **The antinocicep- tive effect of zolpidem and zopiclone in mice.** Pharm Biochem Behav 2005;81:417-23.

- Lin, Shih-Ku. **Rapid detoxification of benzodiazepine or Z-drugs dependence using acetylcholinesterase inhibitors.** S0306-9877(14)00145-5 03/2014

- Pourshams, Maryam and Malakouti, Seyed Kazem. **Zolpidem abuse and dependency in an elderly patient with major depressive disorder: a case report.** Pourshams and Malakouti DARU Journal of Pharmaceutical Sciences 2014.

- Staedt, J Stoppe; Gabriela, G. Hajak; Muller-Struck, A.; Ruther, E. **Schlafstõrungen - Was tun, wenn Schlafmittel nicht mehr helfen? Úbersicht und Fallvorstellung** Psychiatrische Klinik und Poliklinik, Universität Gõttingen Fortsehr. Neurol. Psychiat. 63 (1995) 368-372

- Cavallaro, Roberto; Regazzetti, Maria Grazia; Covelli, Giampiero; Smeraldi, Enrico. **Tolerance and withdrawal with zolpidem**

- Tripodianakis, J.; Potagas, C.; Papageorgiou, P.; Lazaridou, M.; Matikas, N. **Zolpidem-related epileptic seizures: a case report** European Psychiatry 18 (2003) 140-141

- Mariani, John J.; Levin, French R.; **Quetiapine Treatment of Zolpidem Dependence** The American Journal on Addictions, 16:426, 2007

- Benyamina, Amine; Dublanchet, Olivier; Karila, Laurent; Blecha, Lisa; Reynaud, Michel. **Intravenous Zolpidem Abuse: A Case for Serotonin Depletion** The American Journal on Addictions, 16:534, 2007

- Spyridi, Styliani; Diakogiannis, Ioannis; Nimatoudis, Jannis; Iacovides, Apostolos; Kaprinis, Georgios; **Zolpidem dependence in a geriatric patient: a case report.** October 2009-vol. 57, no. 10 letters to the editor

- Ravishankar, Aruna; Carnwath, Tom: **Zolpidem tolerance and dependence: two case reports.** Journal of Psychopharmacology 12(1)

(1998) 103-104

- Chen, Shao-Chien; Chen, Hsi-Chung; Liao, Shih-Cheng; Tseng, Mei-Chih Meg; Lee, Ming-Been; **Detoxification of high-dose zolpidem using cross-titration with an adequate equivalent dose of diazepam.** General Hospital Psychiatry 34 (2012) 210.e5-210.e7

- Sethi, PK; Khandelwal, DC; **Zolpidem at Supratherapeutic Doses can Cause Drug Abuse, Dependence and Withdrawal Seizure.** Japi, vol. 53, february 2005

- Aggarwal, Ashish; Sharma, Dinesh D.; **Zolpidem Withdrawal Delirium: A Case Report.** J Neuropsychiatry Clin Neurosci 22:4, Fali 2010

- Wang, Liang-Jen; Ree, Shao-Chun; Chu, Chin-Lin; Juang, Yeong-Yuh; **Zolpidem dependence and withdrawal seizure - Report of two cases.** Psychiatria Danubina, 2011; Vol. 23, No. 1, pp 76-78

- Djezzar, Samira; Dugarin, Jean; Daily, Sylvain; **Zolpidem and Dextromoramide Abuse with Increased Metabolism.** The American Journal on Addictions, 15: 405- 406, 2006

- Huang, Ming-Chyi; Lin, Hong-Yen; Chen, Chun-Hsin; **Dependence on zolpidem.** Psychiatry and Clinicai Neurosciences (2007), 61,207-208

- Cubala, Wieslaw J.; Landowski, Jerzy; **Seizure following sudden zolpidem withdrawal.** Progress in Neuro-Psychopharmacology & Biological Psychiatry 31 (2007) 539-540

- Liappas, Ioannis A.; Malitas, Petros N.; Dirnopoulos, Nikolaos I; Gitsa, Olympia E.; Liappas, Alexandros I.; Nikolaoul, Chrisoula K.; Christodouloul, Georgios N.; **Three Cases of Zolpidem Dependence Treated with Fluoxetine: The Serotonin Hypothesis.** World J Biol Psychiatry (2003) 4, 93-96

- Quaglioa, GianLuca; Lugobonia, Fabio; Fornasieroa, Anna; Lechib, Alessandra; Gerrac, Gilberto; Mezzelania, Paolo; **Dependence on zolpidem: two case reports of detoxification with flumazenil infusion.** International Clinical Psychopharmacology 2005, Vol 20 No 5

- Golden, Scott A.; Vagnoni, Christopher; Pharm; B.S.; **Zolpidem Dependence and Prescription Fraud.** The American Journal on Addictions 9:96-97, 2000

- Barrero-Hernández, F.J.; Ruiz-Veguilla b, M.; López-López; Casado-Torres, M.L; **Epileptic crises as a manifestation in withdrawal from chronic zolpidem consumption.** Revista neurologia 2002; 34 (3): 253-256

- Krueger, Tillmann HC; Kropp, Stefan; Huber, Thomas J; **High-dose zolpidem dependence in a patient with chronic facial pain.** The Annals of Pharmacotherapy 2005 April, Volume 39 773

- Damm, Julia; Eser, Daniela; Moeller, Hans-Juergen; Rupprecht, Rainer; **Severe dependency on zolpidem in a patient with multiple sclerosis suffering from paraspasticity.** The World Journal of Biological Psychiatry, 2010; 11(2): 516-518

- Imai, Hissei; Matsuishi, Kunitaka; Kitamura, Noboru; Matsui, Yusuke; Tamiya, Satoshi; Tahara, Yumiko; Ishihara, Takashi; Mita, Tatsuo; **Dependence on quetiapine in combination with zolpidem and clonazepam in bipolar depression.** Psychiatry and Clinicai Neurosciences 2009; 63: 426-431

- Kao, Ching-Ling; Huang, Shu-Chi; Yang, Yung-Jen; Tsai, Shih-Jen; **A Case of Parenteral Zolpidem Dependence With Opioid-Like Withdrawal Symptoms. J** Clin Psychiatry 65:9, September 2004

- Rappa, Leonard R; Larose-Pierre, Margareth; Payne, Deidre R;

Eraikhuemen, Nathaniel E; Lanes, Douglas M; Kearson, Margaretta L.; **Detoxification from High- Dose Zolpidem Using Diazepam.** The Annals of Pharmacotherapy 2004 April, Volume 38

- Boulanger-Rostowsky, L.; Fayet, H.; Moussa, N. Bem; Ferrandi, J.; **Dépendance au zolpidem : à propos de deux cas.** L'Encéphale, 2004 ; XXX : 153-5

- Jana, Amlan Kusum; Arora, Manu; Khess, C. R. J.; Praharaj, Samir Kumar; **Case of Zolpidem Dependence Successfully Detoxified with Clonazepam.** The American Journal on Addictions, 17: 343-344, 2008

- Bottlender, R.; Schutz, C.; Moller, H. J.; Soyka, M.; **Zolpidem Dependence in a Patient with Former Polysubstance Abuse** Pharmacopsychiat. 30 (1997) 108

- Gilhert, Donald L.; Staats, Peter S.; **Seizure Ater Withdrawal From Supratherapeutic Doses of Zolpidem Tartrate. A Selective Omega I Benzodiazepine Receptor Agonist.** Journal of Pain and Symptom Management Vol 14 n°3 August 1997

- Sakkas, P.; Psarros, C.; Masdrakis, V.; Liappas, J.; Christodoulou, G.N. **Dependence on zolpidem: a case report.** Eur Psychiatry 1999 ; 14 : 358-9

- Svitek, Jana ; Heberlein, Annemarie; Bleich, Stefan; Wiltfang, Jens; Kornhuber, Johannes; Hillemacher, Thomas; **Extensive craving in high dose zolpidem dependence.** Progress in Neuro-Psychopharmacology & Biological Psychiatry 32 (2008) 591-592

- Quaglio, Gianluca; Faccini, Marco; Vigneau, Caroline Victorri; Casari, Rebecca; Mathewson, Sophie; Licata, Manuela; Lugoboni, Fabio; **Megadose Bromazepam and Zolpidem Dependence: Two Case Reports of Treatment with Flumazenil and Valproate** Substance Abuse, 33:195-198, 2012

- Keuroghlian, Alex S.; Barry, Alan S.; Weiss, Roger D.; **Circadian Dysregulation, Zolpidem Dependence, and Withdrawal Seizure in a Resident Physician Performing Shift Work.** The American Journal on Addictions, 00:1-2, 2012

- Bhatia, Manjeet S.; Kohli, Gurdeet S.; **Iatrogenic Zolpidem Dependence.** J Neuropsychiatry Clin Neurosci 26:2, Spring 2014

- Gericke, Christian A. ; Ludolph, Albert C. **Chronic Abuse of Zolpidem.** JAMA, december 1994,-vol 272, n°22

- Ware JC, Walsh JK, Scharf MB, Roehrs T, Roth T, Vogel GW. **Minimal rebound insomnia after treatment with 10-mg zolpidem.** Clin Neuropharmacol. 1997 Apr;20(2):116-25.

- Alves, H., Kessler, F., & Ratto, L. R. C. (2004). **Comorbidity: alcohol use and other psychiatric disorders.** Revista Brasileira de Psiquiatria, 26(1), 51-53.

- Scheffer, M., Pasa, G. G., & de Almeida, R. M. M. (2010). **Alcohol, cocaine and crack cocaine dependence and psychiatric disorders.** Psicologia: Teoria e Pesquisa, 26(3), 533-541.

- Zaleski, M., Laranjeira, R. R., Marques, A. C. P. R., Ratto, L., Romano, M., Alves, N. P., & Lemos, T. (2006). **Guidelines of the Brazilian Association for the Study of Alcohol and Other Drugs (Associação Brasileira Comorbidades psiquiátricas em dependentes químicos).**

(ABEAD) for the diagnosis and treatment of psychiatric comorbidities and alcohol and other substance dependence. Brazilian Journal of Psychiatry, 28, 142-148

- Laranjeira, Ronaldo and collaborators; **Chemical dependency prevention, treatment and public policies,** 2011;

- Diagnostic and Statistical Manual of Mental Disorders - DSM-5;

CHAPTER 8

Table 1 legend

1- **Restlessness**; severe agitation, crying, severe anxiety, impatience, loss of energy, insomnia, irritability, verbal aggression, distraction, increased appetite, physical symptoms such as headaches and dizziness, trembling, and **increased desire for a higher dosage of opium;**
2-**Great convulsive** disorder;
3-Anxiety, palpitation, tremor;
4-Anxious **mood**, global insomnia and restlessness, facial spasm, mouth opening, **convulsion**, clouded consciousness, psychomotor retardation, regressed attitude and behaviour, disorientation to time maintained for the following 5 days;
5-**Insomnia**, anxiety, palpitations and dyspnoea. The following day, disturbance of consciousness, facial spasm, mouth opening, protrusion of tongue and limbs, **convulsions** for about 3 minutes. The EEG carried out revealed epileptic peaks of discharge and of great misdiagnosis;
6-**History** of violence and agitation; behaviour, not recognising others, irritability, and irrelevant speech 2 days before;
7-**Anxiety**, hand tremor, sweating and palpitations, **convulsions**;
8-**Tremor**, sweating, nausea, irritability, anger and psychomotor agitation;
9-**Depression**, moodiness, irritability, anxiety and perplexity, headache.
10-**Tremors**, sweating, chills and headache.
11-**Convulsion**, opisthotonus, oculogyric crisis;
12-**Confusion**, amnesia, **convulsion**;
13-**Agitation**, tremor, sweating, tachycardia and three episodes of **seizures;**
14-**Anxiety**, dysthymic mood, irritability, lack of energy, difficulty concentrating;
15-**Low** mood with suicidal ideas, psychomotor retardation, lack of concentration and apparent time disorientation.
16-**Anxiety**, panic attacks, feeling of being watched;

Article reference	**Age**	**Gender Male (M) Female (F)**	**Psychiatric Comorbidity**	**Initial dose (mg)**	**Final dose (mg)**	**Withdrawal symptoms**	**Time of use**	**Medications used / dose MG**	**Pharmaceutical measures**	**Treatment time. D(days) S(weeks) M(months)**	**Treatment regime. Hospital (H) Outpatient(A)**
01)Pourshams, Maryam and Malakouti, Seyed Kazem; 2014	62	F	Depression / opioid dependence	10	570	1 (seizure)	2 years	Gabapentin 900 trazodone 100 Sertraline 200 Methadone 40	-	3 S + 2 M	H A
02) Lin, Shih-Ku, 2014	48	F	depression	--	400	-	3 years	Galantamine 2x 16 mg for 3 days Trazodone 100	-	3 M	-

								Quetiapine 50 Flunitrazepam 60			
03) Manjeet S. Bhatia, M.B.B.S.; Gurdeet S. Kohli, M.B.B.S.; 2014	48	F	THB	-	400/500	-	15 months	Mirtazapine 30	-	8 S	-
04) Keuroghlian, Alex S. et al 2012	34	M	THB / alcohol and opioid abuser	100	400	2 (seizure)	2,5 years	Chlordiazepox. Zolpidem 30=>20=>10 => discount (3 days)	Psychotherapy. AA	3 D	H
05) Quaglio, Gianluca MD *et al 2012*	39	M	Depression and OCD anxiety	-	400 a 1800	-	15 years	Flumazenil 0.5 mg continuous 1st day; 1mg 2nd day; clonazepam for 4 days (6=>4=>2=>1)	-	11 D + 3 S	H
06)Chen, Shao-Chien et al, 2011	53	F	Depression / substance abuse	10	100 a 160 160 + More 100	3	4 years	**1ª hospitalisation** Sertraline 100 Quetiapine 25 Clonazepam 3 Flunitrazepam 2 **2nd hospitalisation** Clonazepam 0.25 Clonazepam 3 Paroxetine 40 Quetiapine 25 Flunitrazepam 2.5	-	2M 2 D 3 S 3 D 1 M 3 D=>1 M	H

								3ª hospitalisation Cross-exchange: zolpidem 10 diazepam 5 Diazepam 50 Diazepam 5 Paroxetine 60 Flunitrazepam 1			
07)Wang, Liang-Jen et al 2011	43	F	dysthymia	50 a 60	200 a 400	4 (seizure)	2 years	Lorazepam 2 alprazolam 0.5	-	-	H
07) Wang, Liang-Jen et al 2011	35	F	Depression Abuse of hypnotics and analgesics	10 a 20	400 a 500	5 (seizure)	1 year	clonazepam	-	-	H
08) Aggarwal, Ashish et al , 2010	62	M	Headache / depression	10	160 a 180	6	2 years	Cross-exchange with clonazepam Topiramate 200 Paroxetine 25 Flunarezine 10	-	-	H A
09) Damm, Julia et al, 2010	49	F	Multiple sclerosis and paraspasticity	10	700 a 800	yes (no description)	8 years	Diazepam 40 Doxepin 150 Carbamaz. 400 Tolperison (paraspasticity) 100	-	-	H
10) Spyridi, Styliani, 2009	78	M	Depend. On benzod.	10	200	yes (no description)	-	Cross-exchange Zolpidem 200 mirtazapine 30 ac. Valproic 500 => reduced zolpidem increased mirtazapine 45 and ac. Valproic 1000	-	40 D	H

								quetiapine 50 => 100 when removing zolpidem			
11) Chen, Chun-Yen, et al 2009	9	5 F	THB	-	600	3	-	Valproic acid 1000 Mirtazapine 60 Clozapine 150 Clonazepam 4 Midazolam 15	-	3 S	H
12) Jana, Amlan Kusum, 2008	3	3 M	Hist. Opioid dependence, smoking	-	150	4 (seizure)	3 years	Clonazepam 4	-	-	H
13) Svitek J et al 2008	7	2 M	smoking and alcohol consumption	--	800	7 (seizure)	-	300 zolpidem/ 900 carbamazepine		3 S	H
14) Benyamine, Amine et al , 2007	2	2 F	Heroin and other drugs	30/40 **EV**	50 **EV**	-	-	Paroxetine 40mg	-	-	-
15) Mariani, John J. et al 2007	2	5 M	Heroin and other drug addiction / insomnia	10	250	yes (no description)	6 months	Clonazepam (withdrawal) Trazodone 200 (unsuccessful) Gabapentin (unsuccessful) Quetiapine 800	-	5 D	H A A A
16) HUANG, MING-CHYI et al 2006	4	3 F	adjustment disorder, dysthymia	10 a 20	100 0 => 120 0 => 200 0	4 (seizure)	2 years	Diazepam 20 Trazodone 100	-	10 D	H
17)Djezzar, Samira et al, 2006	8	3 M	Dep. Dextromoramide / methadone	-	800	7 (seizure)	-	Zolpidem 40 benzodiazepines	-	-	H
18) Cubala, Wieslaw	9	2 F	Insomnia (history of trans.	5 a 10	160	7 (seizure)	2 years	Divalproate 900	-	-	H

J. et al 2006			dissociative depression)								
19) Quaglio, GianLuca et al 2005	38	M	Multiple drug dependence	10 a 20	700 / 900	8	6 months	Flumasenil 0.5 => 1 Clobazam 10 mg Sertraline 100	-	-	H
19) Quaglio, GianLuca et al 2005	27	M	Anxiety and panic History of experimenting with various drugs	-	1600	-	6 months	Flumasenil 0.5=> 1 Clonazepam 2 Clobazam 10 Haloperidol Baclofen (craving) sertraline	-	-	H
20) PK Sethi, DC Khandelwal et al 2005 JAPI - VOL. 53 - FEBRUARY 2005	42	M	Panic on the flight	10	200	7 (seizure)	2 years	Phenytoin 300 Zolpidem 20 (reduced to high)	-	-	H
21) Krueger, Tillmann HC et al 2004	39	F	Facial pain; history of drug use, benzodiazepines, barbiturates;	10	600	7 (seizure)	2 years	Oxazepam 20 mg for 4 days + carbamazepine 200 for 3 days	-	10 D	H
22) Kao, Ching-Ling et al 2004	35	M	History of drug use (injecting heroin)	10	400 **EV**	-	1 year	Lormetazepam 1.5	-	3 S	H
23)L. Boulanger-Rostowsky, et al 2004	30	M	T.P. BORDER MULTIP. DRUGS			9		Paroxetine, diazepam, risperidone			H
24)Rappa, Leonard R et al 2004	46	M	History of drug use	5	400	10	2 years	Diazepam 10 Atenolol 50 Nefazodone 100=>600	-	7 days	H

25) Tripodianaki, J. et al 2003	4 3	F	Depression / insomnia	-	600	11	6 months	Diazepam 30 Phenytoin 500	-		H
26) loannis A. Liappas et al World J Biol Psychiatry (2003) 4, 93 - 96	3 0	M	History of cocaine use Smoker	-	200 / 300	-	-	Fluoxetine 40	CBT	-	-
26) loannis A. Liappas et al World J Biol Psychiatry (2003) 4, 93 - 96	4 2	M	Insomnia	10	300	12 (seizure)	3 years	Fluoxetine 40	-	-	H
26) loannis A. Liappas et al World J Biol Psychiatry (2003) 4, 93 - 96	3 5	F	Onicofagia; trasnt. Food; Anxiety; trans. Mood; Initial insomnia	-	100 / 150	-	3 months	Fluoxetine 40	CBT	-	-
27) Barrero-Hernández, F.J. et al 2002	5 0	F	Mild depression; trans. Adaptive	-	450	13 (seizure)	-	Fluoxetine lorazepam	-	-	H
28) Golden, Scott A., et al 2000	3 9	M	-	10	40	yes (no description)	7 months	Chlordiazepox.	-	-	-
29) P. Sakkas, et al 1999	4 4	F	History of addiction to drugs / depression	10	100 / 300	14 (seizure)	2 years	Clorazepate 30; Fluoxetine 60;	-	-	H

								zolpidem 20 (in reduction)			
30) Ravishankar, Aruna et al 1998	55	F	depression	-	200	15	2,5 years	diazepam	-	-	-
30) Ravishankar, Aruna et al 1998	28	M	-	-	100	16	-	zolpidem in gradual reduction	-	-	-
31) Gilhert, Donald L., et al 1997	37	M	-	10	130	7 (seizure)	-	diazepam	-	-	H
32) Bottlender, R., et al 1997	53	M	History of multi-drug use Drugs / parkinsonism	15	140			Zolpidem gradual withdrawal		5 days	H
33) Staedt, J, et al 1995	45	M	-	10	30	-	-	Trimipramine 100	-	-	A
34) Cavallero, Roberto et al 1991	31	F	Depression / residual insomnia	20	70 / 80	3 (myoclonus)	super. a 2 months	Diazepam 40 mg Zolpidem gradual withdrawal	-	1 M	A
34) Cavallero, Roberto et al 1991	60	F	Trans. Pers. Histrionic and paranoid	10	100	7 (seizure)	super. 2 months	Clonazepam 2	-	3 days	H

F10-F19 Mental and behavioural disorders due to psychoactive substance use

This group comprises numerous disorders that differ in their severity and diverse symptoms, but which have in common the fact that they are all attributed to the use of one or more psychoactive substances, whether or not prescribed by a doctor. The third character of the code identifies the substance involved and the fourth character specifies the clinical picture. The codes should be used, as determined, for each substance specified, but it should be noted that not all fourth character codes can be applied to all substances.

The identification of the psychoactive substance must be based on all possible sources of information. This includes: information provided by the subject themselves, analyses of blood and other body fluids, characteristic physical and psychological symptoms, clinical signs and behaviours, and other evidence such as drugs found on the patient and reports from well-informed third parties. Many drug users consume more than one type of psychoactive substance. The main diagnosis should be categorised, if possible, according to the toxic substance or category of toxic substances that is most responsible for the clinical picture or

determines its essential characteristics. Additional diagnoses should be coded when other drugs or categories of drugs have been consumed in sufficient quantities to cause intoxication (fourth common character .0), adverse health effects (fourth common character .1), dependence (fourth common character .2) or other disorders (fourth common character .3-.9).
The diagnosis of multiple substance use disorders (F19.-) should only be reserved for cases where the choice of drugs is made in a chaotic and indiscriminate manner, or in those cases where the contributions of different drugs are mixed.

Excludes:

abuse of non-dependent substances (F55)

The following fourth-character subdivisions must be used with categories F10-F19:

F13 - Mental and behavioural disorders due to the use of sedatives and hypnotics

.0 Acute poisoning

A state resulting from the use of a psychoactive substance and comprising disturbances in consciousness, cognitive faculties, perception, affect or behaviour, or other psycho-physiological functions and responses. The disturbances are directly related to the acute pharmacological effects of the substance consumed, and disappear over time, with complete healing, except in cases where organic lesions or other complications have arisen. Complications include: trauma, aspiration of vomit, delirium, coma, convulsions and other medical complications. The nature of these complications depends on the pharmacological category of the substance consumed as well as its mode of administration.
SOE drunkenness
Trance and possession states in psychoactive substance intoxication
Acute alcohol intoxication
Pathological intoxication intoxication meaning poisoning (T36-T50)
47

1 Use harmful to health

Consumption of a psychoactive substance that is harmful to health. Complications can be physical (for example, hepatitis as a result of injections of the drug by the person themselves) or psychological (for example, depressive episodes secondary to heavy alcohol consumption).

Abuse of a psychoactive substance

2 Dependency syndrome

A set of behavioural, cognitive and physiological phenomena that develop after repeated consumption of a psychoactive substance, typically associated with a powerful desire to take the drug, difficulty in controlling consumption, persistent use despite its harmful consequences, greater priority given to drug use over other activities and obligations, an increase in tolerance for the drug and sometimes a state of physical withdrawal.
Dependency syndrome can concern a specific psychoactive substance (for example, smoking, alcohol or diazepam), a category of psychoactive substances (for example, opiates) or a wider range of pharmacologically different substances.

Chronic alcoholism
Dipsomania
Toxicomania

3 Withdrawal syndrome

A set of symptoms, grouped in different ways and varying in severity, that occur during absolute or relative abstinence from a psychoactive substance consumed over a long period of time. The onset and evolution of the withdrawal syndrome are limited in time and depend on the category and dose of the substance consumed immediately before stopping or reducing consumption. The withdrawal syndrome can be complicated by seizures.

4 Withdrawal syndrome with delirium

State in which the withdrawal syndrome as defined in the fourth character .3 is complicated by the occurrence of delirium, according to the criteria in F05.-. This condition can also include convulsions. When organic factors are also considered in its aetiology, the condition should be classified under F05.8.

Delirium tremens (alcohol-induced)

5 Psychotic disorder

A set of psychotic phenomena that occur during or immediately after the consumption of a psychoactive substance, but which cannot be explained entirely on the basis of acute intoxication and which do not also form part of a withdrawal syndrome. The state is characterised by the presence of hallucinations (typically auditory, but often polysensory), distortion of perceptions, delusional ideas (often of the paranoid or persecutory type), psychomotor disturbances (agitation or stupor) and abnormal affections, which can range from intense fear to ecstasy. The senses are not usually impaired, but there may be a certain degree of cloudiness of consciousness, although confusion may be present, but it is not serious.

"Bad trips" (drugs)

Excludes:

Hallucinos 1
is

Jealousy alcoholic
Paranoia

SOE psychosis J

Excludes:

psychotic disorders induced by alcohol or other psychoactive substances, residual or of late onset (F10-F19 with common fourth character .7)

.6 Amnesic syndrome

Syndrome dominated by the presence of significant chronic memory disorders (recent and old facts). Immediate memory is usually preserved and memory of recent events is typically more disturbed than remote memory. There are usually manifest disturbances in temporal orientation and the chronology of events, as well as difficulties in learning new information. The syndrome can present intense confabulation, but this may not be present in all cases. Other cognitive functions are generally relatively well preserved and amnesic deficits are disproportionate to other disorders.

Psychosis or Korsakov syndrome, induced by alcohol or another psychoactive substance or unspecified

Alcohol- or drug-induced amnesic disorder

Excludes:

psychosis or non-alcoholic Korsakov syndrome (F04)

.7 Residual or late-onset psychotic disorder

A disorder in which alcohol- or psychoactive substance-induced changes in cognition, affect, personality or behaviour persist beyond the period during which they can be considered a direct effect of the substance. The occurrence of the disorder must be directly linked to the consumption of a psychoactive substance. Cases in which the first manifestations occur clearly later than the episode(s) of drug use should only be coded under this character where there is evidence to unequivocally attribute the manifestations to the residual effect of the substance. Flashbacks can be differentiated from a psychotic state, partly because they are episodic and often of very short duration, and partly because they reproduce previous experiences linked to alcohol or psychoactive substances. Dementia:

1 alcoholic SOE

2 and other mild forms of long-term cognitive impairment

"Flashbacks

Chronic cerebral syndrome of alcoholic origin

Disorder (of) (of):

3 residual affective
4 persistent perceptions induced by the use of hallucinogens
5 personality and residual behaviour
6 late-onset psychosis induced by the use of psychoactive substances

Excludes:

alcohol- or psychoactive substance-induced psychotic state (F10-F19 with common fourth character .5)
Korsakov syndrome, alcohol or psychoactive substance induced (F10-F19 with fourth common character .6)

.8 Other mental or behavioural disorders

.9 Mental or behavioural disorder not otherwise specified

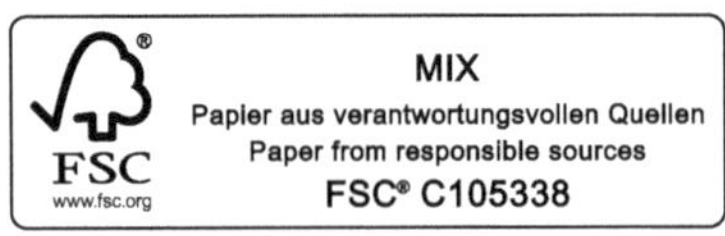

Printed by Books on Demand GmbH, Norderstedt / Germany